Knee Replacement 101

Susan Yovanno

To Kate

CONTENTS

Disclaimer

The intention of this book is to provide helpful information on the subjects discussed. The information contained herein should not be used as a substitute for medical advice from a qualified physician or other licensed health care provider. For diagnosis or treatment of any medical problem, consult your physician. The publisher and author are not responsible for any specific healthcare needs that may require medical supervision and are not liable for any damages or negative consequences from any action or application of any material in this book.

ACKNOWLEDGMENTS

Thank you to Sandbase Studios and Sprout Creatives.

1 PREP YOURSELF

The healthier you are going in to surgery, the better your outcome. To prepare yourself for knee replacement surgery, you can work on knee range of motion, leg strength, flexibility, balance, and optimal body mass.

Exercises to improve **range of motion**:

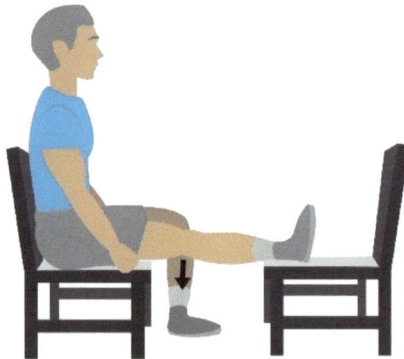

Knee Extension. Prop your foot on a chair in front of you, and let your knee hang for a gravity assisted extension stretch. To increase the stretch, alternate leaning your trunk forward, pressing down with your knee, or pulling your toes toward you. Let knee hang 5-10 minutes, 2x/day.
* Normal knee extension (straight) is 0 degrees.

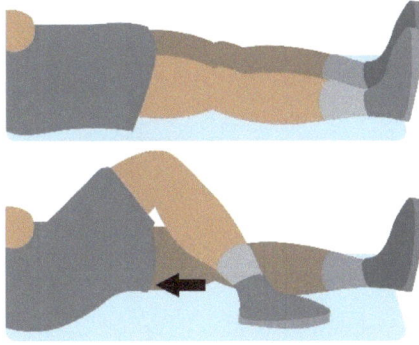

Knee flexion. Lying on your back, slide your heel toward your bottom, hold for several seconds, then return to start position. Perform 15 repetitions, 2x/day.
*Normal knee flexion (bend) is ~ 135 degrees depending on age and body type

Exercises to improve **strength**:

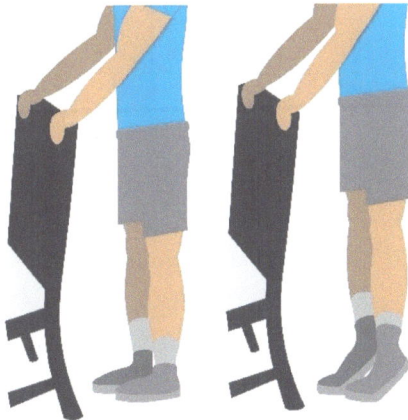

Heel Raises. Hold onto a stable surface for balance, rise up on your toes. Perform 15 repetitions, 2-3x/day.

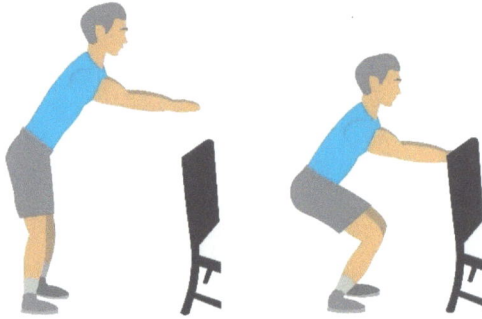

Partial Squats. Hold onto a stable surface for balance, partially squat down as if you are going to sit in a chair, then rise to start position. Perform 10-15 repetitions, 2x/day.

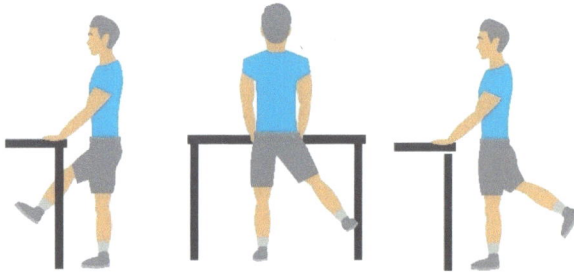

Hip 3 ways. Holding onto stable surface for balance. Stand up straight, raise the straight to the front, side, and back. Perform 10 repetitions in each direction, 2x/day. Add cuff weights or resisted bands at the ankle as needed for progression.

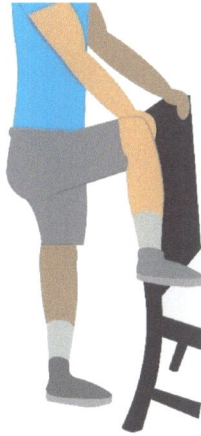

High March. Hold onto a stable surface for balance.
Raise the knee toward your chest, into a high march
position. Perform 10 repetitions, 2x/day.

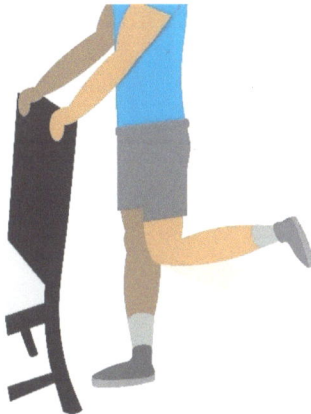

Hamstring Curls. Hold onto stable surface for balance.
Raise foot toward your bottom bending the knee. Perform
15 repetitions, 2x/day.

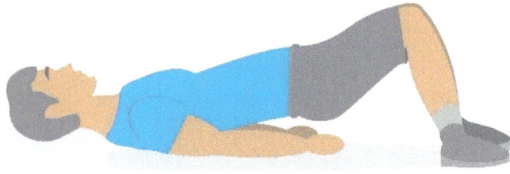

Bridging. Lie on your back, squeeze your gluteals, and raise your bottom toward the ceiling. Hold 3 seconds, return to start position. Perform 10 repetitions, 2x/day.

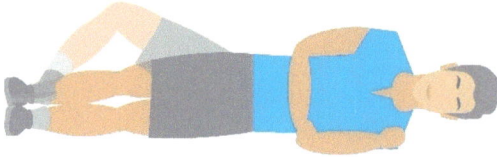

Clams. Lie on your side with your pelvis vertical. Using your gluteal muscles, raise your knee toward the ceiling while keeping your feet together. Keep your pelvis slightly forward. Perform 15 repetitions, 2x/day.

Exercises to improve **flexibility**:

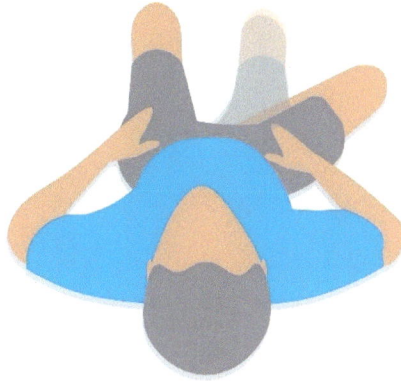

Hip Rotator Stretch. Lie on your back with your knees bent. Let your knee gently fall out to the side. Your pelvis should stay flat on table. Hold 15 seconds. Perform 3 repetitions, 2x/day.

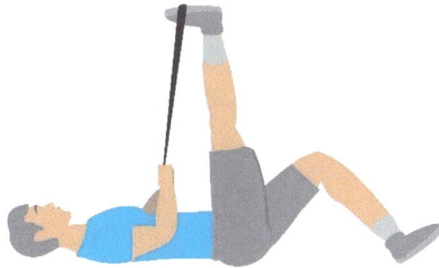

Hamstring Stretch. Lie on your back, raise your leg in straight position with a strap, leash, or belt. Hold 15 seconds. Perform 3 repetitions, 2x/day.

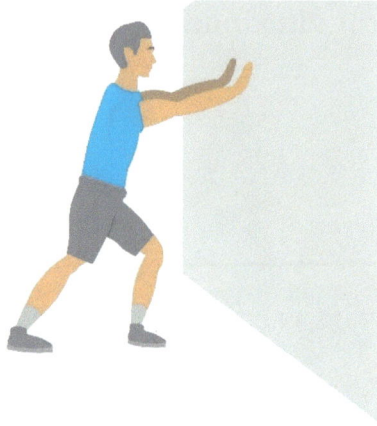

Calf stretch. Standing with toes pointing straight ahead, take a step forward, hands on wall for balance. Keep heel down, lean forward until a stretch is felt in the calf muscle. Hold for 15 seconds. Perform 3 repetitions, 2x/day.

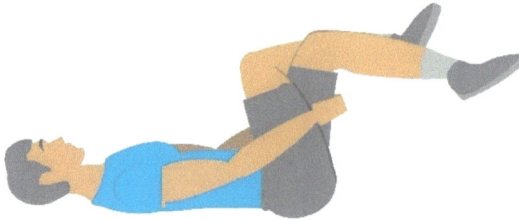

Piriformis Stretch. Lie on your back and cross one leg over other, pull legs toward chest. Hold for 15 seconds. Perform 3 repetitions, 2x/day.

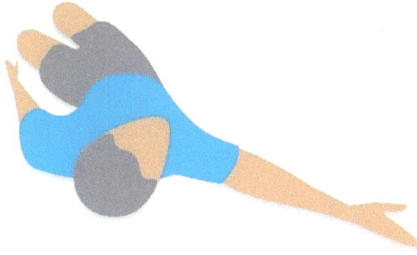

Open Book Stretch. Lie on your side with your hips and knees flexed. Extend the top arm toward the ceiling, rotate shoulders to lie flat while watching the moving hand. Perform 10 repetitions, 2x/day.

Exercises to improve **balance**:

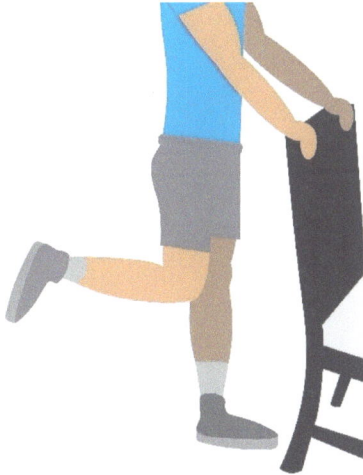

Single Leg Stance. Hold onto stable surface for balance. Lift one leg from the floor, and balance on the stance leg. Push down with the big toe of the stance leg and contract the gluteal and abdominal muscles. Hold 15 seconds. Perform 3 repetitions, 1x/day.
* Progress from tight grip with hands to light grip to fingertip touch as able

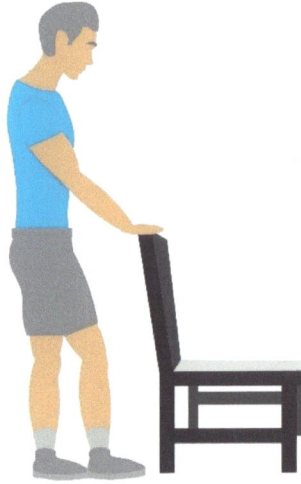

Tandem Stance. Hold onto stable surface for balance.
Stand with the toes of one foot touching the heel of the
other foot. Push down with the big toes and contract the
gluteal and abdominal muscles. Hold 15 seconds. Switch
foot position and repeat. Perform 3 repetitions, 1x/day.
*Progress from tight grip with hands to light grip, to
fingertip touch as able

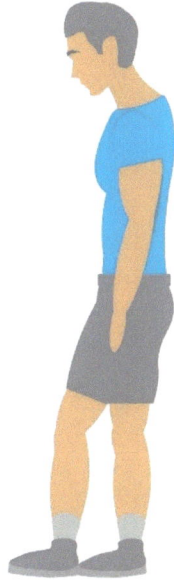

Tandem Walk. Use kitchen counter for balance. Walk a straight line of 10 feet with the toes of one foot touching the heel of the other foot. Perform 3 repetitions, 1x/day.

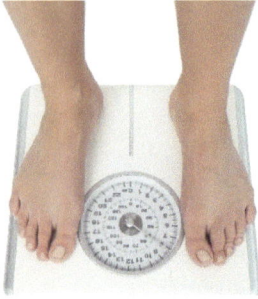

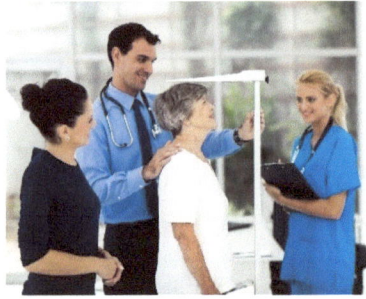

Body Mass Index or BMI. BMI is a measure of body fat based on height and weight.

BMI formula: your weight in pounds divided by (your height in inches x your height in inches) x 703.

Example for a 150lb, 5'4" person: 150 divided by (64 x 64) x 703 = 25.7

BMI categories:

Underweight	Below 18.5
Normal	18.5 - 24.9
Overweight	25.0 - 29.9
Obesity	30.0 and above

A diet of fruits, vegetables, and light protein combined with 30 minutes of daily exercise or physical activity will promote optimal body mass. Decreasing dietary fat and carbohydrates will decrease caloric intake which can help lower blood pressure and blood glucose, as well as improve cholesterol levels. Walking, aquatic exercise, stationary cycling, and yoga are good options for those with joint pain.

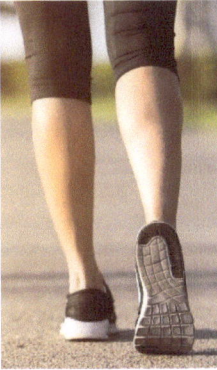

Walking

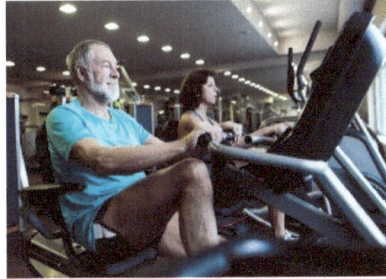

Cycling

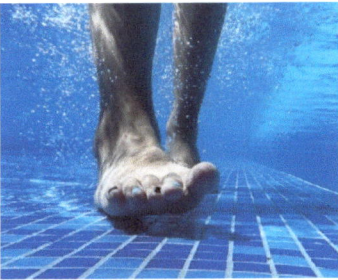

Aquatic Exercise

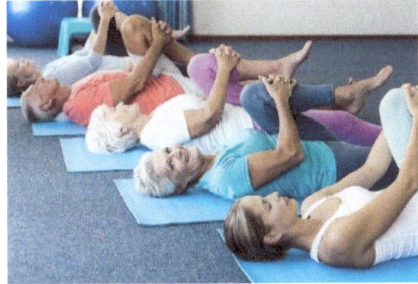

Yoga

Stop Smoking. Aside from damaging your respiratory system, smoking damages the circulatory system. Nicotine in cigarettes, gum, and electronic devices comprises capillary blood flow.

2 PREP YOUR HOME

Preparing your home prior to knee replacement surgery, will be beneficial for your mobility around the home, and for fall prevention. As stairs may be difficult initially, setting up a temporary first floor bedroom is optimal. You will be using a walker initially; removal of throw rugs, extension cords, and any other floor clutter is recommended. Small pets can present a tripping hazard; plan to use extra caution if they will be in or around your walking area. Ensure any railings or grab bars you have are sturdy. Install grab rails as needed. Height-adjustable commode chairs are beneficial for bathroom use, and night-time bedroom use. A shower chair or bench can ease getting in/out of shower or tub area, and is beneficial for those who cannot tolerate prolonged standing while bathing. Handheld shower hoses can be useful for water control. Cold packs and/or an ice machine can be used for swelling management after surgery.

*Consider a stay in a rehabilitation facility if returning home post-operatively is not optimal.

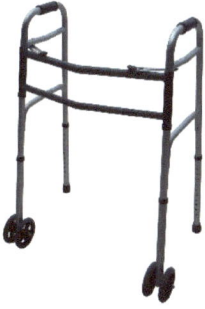

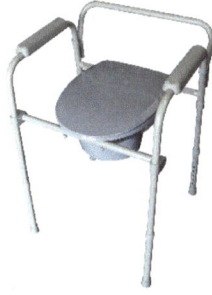

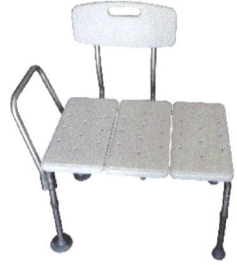

Front wheel
walker

Height-adjustable
commode chair

Shower bench

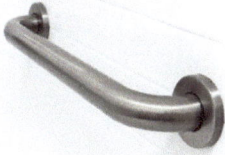

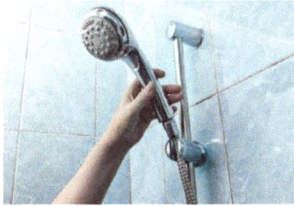

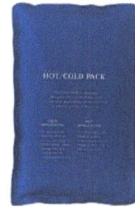

Grab Rail

Handheld shower
hose

Cold Pack

3 POST-OP EXERCISES

Exercises to perform upon waking from surgery until you leave the hospital:

Ankle Pumps.   Elevate the leg above your heart using pillows or hospital bed.   Pump the foot up and down (point and flex.) Perform 15 repetitions, 3x/day.

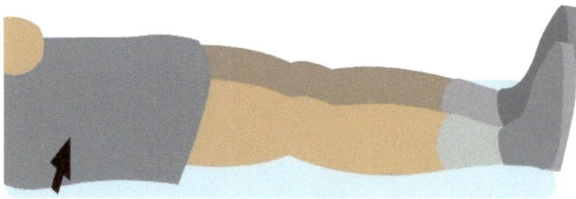

Gluteal Set. Tighten/squeeze your buttock muscles. Hold 5 seconds. Perform 10 repetitions, 3x/day.

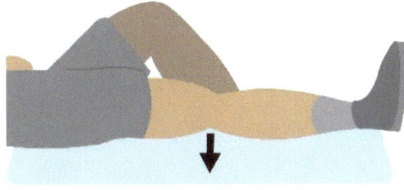

Quadricep Set. Tighten the thigh muscle, push the back of the knee down to straighten the leg. Hold 5 seconds. Perform 10 repetitions, 3x/day.

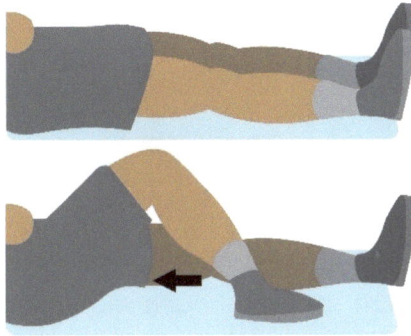

Heel Slide. Slide the foot up toward your bottom, hold 3 seconds, then return to start position. Perform 15 repetitions, 2x/day.

4 HOME EXERCISES

Exercises to perform at home:

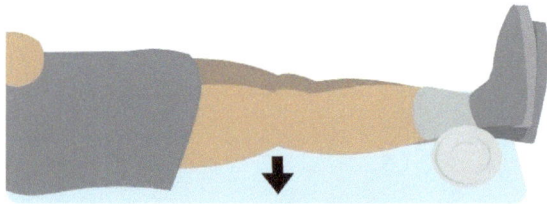

Quad Set. Place a small towel roll under your ankle. Tighten your thigh muscle, push down with your knee. Hold 5 seconds. Perform 10 repetitions, 3x/day.

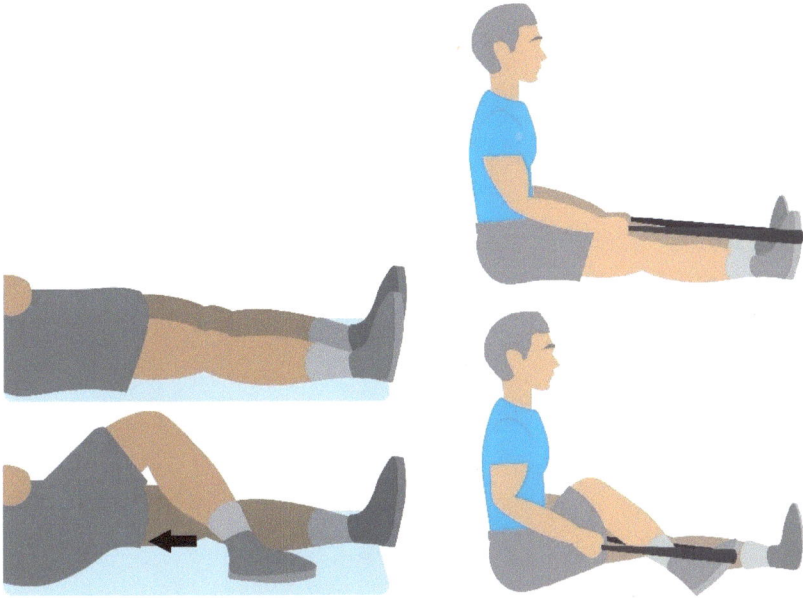

Heel Slides and **Heel Slides with Strap**. Slide your foot toward your bottom using your own muscle power, use a strap, leash, or belt around the foot to pull knee into increased bend position. Hold 5 seconds. Perform 10 repetitions, 3x/day.

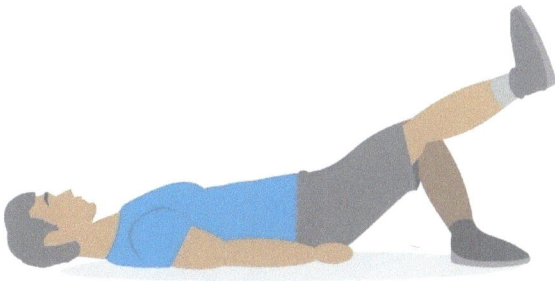

Straight Leg Raise. Pull foot toward your head, tighten thigh muscle, raise leg to the height of the opposite knee. Hold for 3-5 seconds. Perform 10 repetitions, 2x/day.

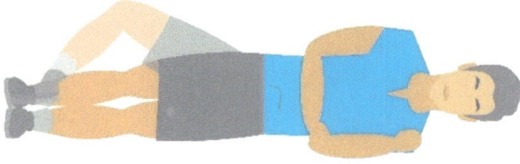

Clamshells. Lie on your side with hips and knees bent. Raise upper knee toward ceiling, while keeping feet together. Hold for 3 seconds. Perform 15 repetitions, 2x/day.

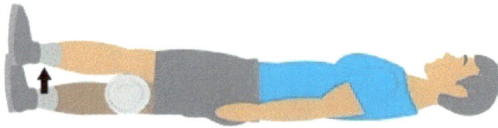

Short Arc Quad. Lie on your back with a rolled pillow under the knee. Pull your foot toward your head, straighten the leg while keeping your knee on the pillow. Hold for 5 seconds. Perform 10 repetitions, 2x/day.

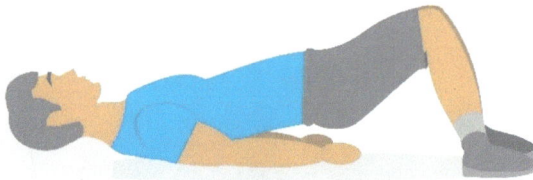

Bridging. Squeeze the gluteal muscles and raise your bottom toward the ceiling. Hold 5 seconds, return to start position. Perform 15 repetitions, 2x/day.

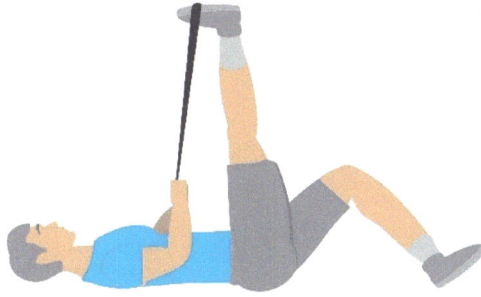

Hamstring Stretch. Using a strap, leash, or belt looped around the foot, raise the leg until a stretch is felt in the back of the thigh and knee. Hold 15 seconds. Perform 3 repetitions, 2x/day.

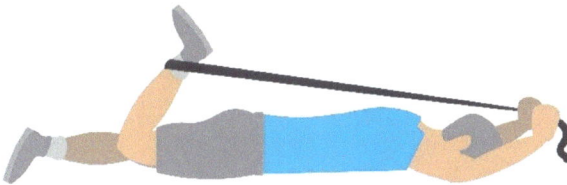

Quadriceps Stretch. Lie on your stomach. Use a strap, leash, or belt, pull the ankle towards your bottom. Hold 10 seconds. Perform 3 repetitions, 2x/day.
*do not perform this exercise if you cannot tolerate the prone position or have difficulty getting strap in place

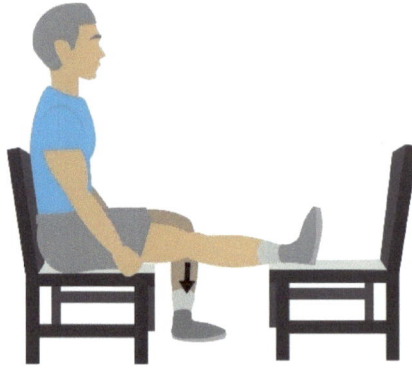

Quad Set with chair. Place your ankle on a chair in front of you. Tighten the thigh muscle, push your down knee to straighten the leg. Hold 5 seconds. Perform 10 repetitions, 3x/day.

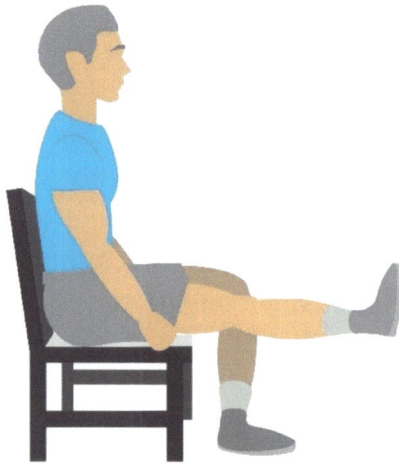

Long Arc Quad. Sitting in a chair, pull the foot toward your head and raise the lower leg until the knee is straight. Hold 3 seconds. Perform 15 repetitions 2x/day.

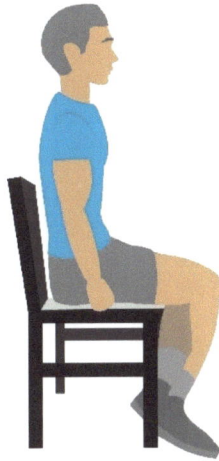

Knee Flexion Stretch in Sitting. Slide the foot of the knee replacement leg under your chair. Use your other leg to push into further bending of the knee. Hold 10 seconds. Perform 3 repetitions, 2x/day.

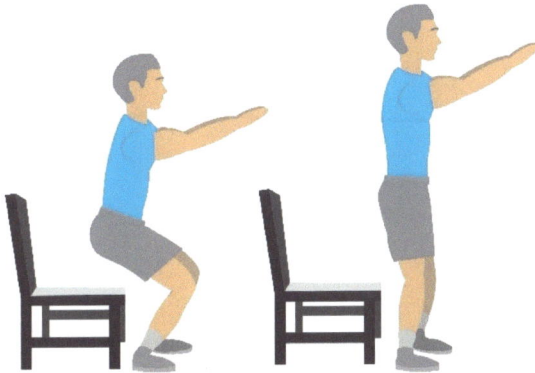

Sit to stand. From seated position, scoot toward edge of seat, lean forward and rise to stand. Use hands as needed to push off. Perform 5 - 10 repetitions, 2x/day.

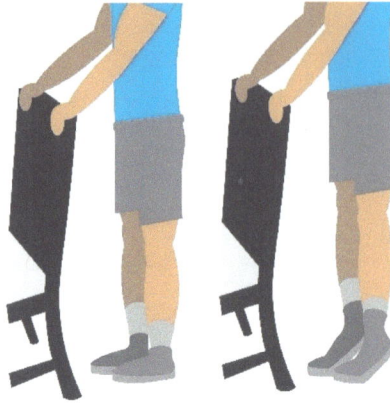

Heel Raises. Hold stable surface for balance. Stand with toes pointed forward, raise heels from floor. Perform 15 repetitions, 2x/day.

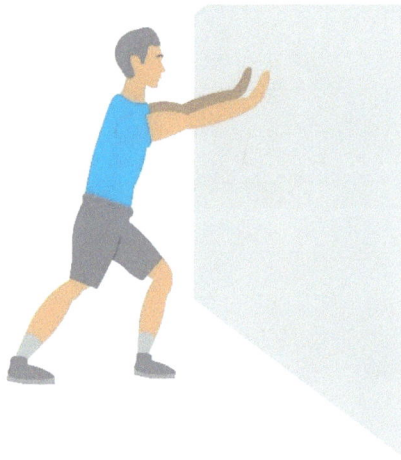

Calf Stretch. In standing with toes pointed forward, take a step forward and lean forward until a stretch is felt in the calf of the leg behind. Hold 15 seconds. Perform 3 repetitions, 2x/day.

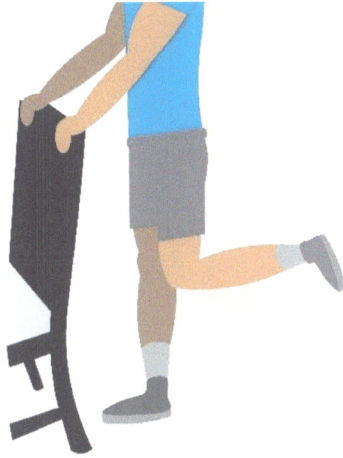

Hamstring Curls. Pull foot toward bottom, bending knee. Perform 15 repetitions, 2x/day.

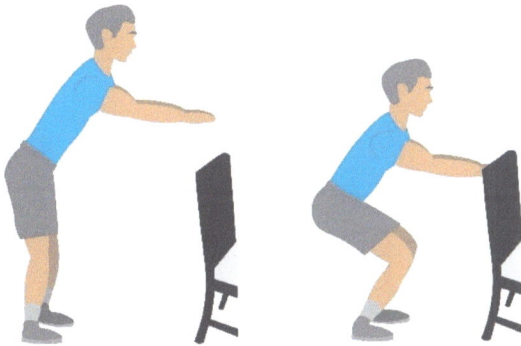

Partial Squats. Holding onto stable surface for balance, partially squat as if you were to sit in a chair. Perform 10 repetitions, 2x/day.

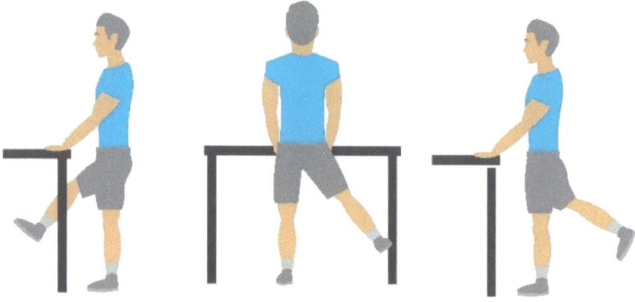

Hip 3 ways. Holding onto stable surface for balance. Standing up straight, raise the straight to the front, side, and back. Perform 10 repetitions in each direction, 2x/day. *Add cuff weights or resisted bands at the ankle as needed for progression

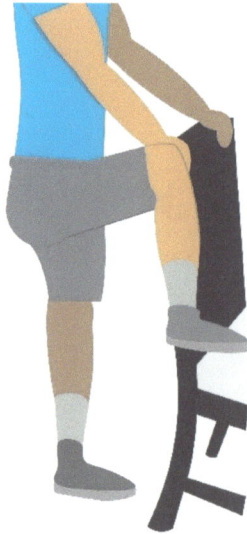

High March. Hold onto stable surface for balance. Stand up straight, raise knee toward ceiling. Perform 10 repetitions, 2x/day.

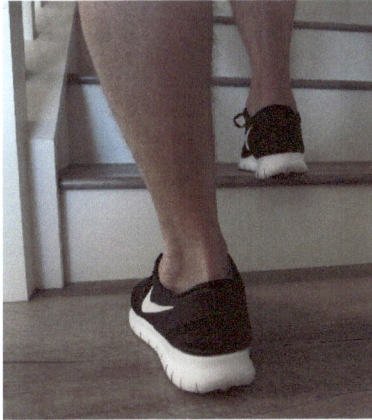

Step Ups. Lean forward slightly, step up, step down. Repeat leading with other leg. Perform 10 repetitions, 2x/day.

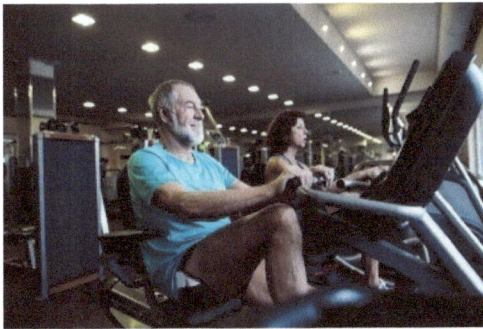

Stationary Bike. Pedal a recumbent or upright stationary bike. Initially pedal partial revolutions (forward/back), until you can complete a full revolution. Perform 10 minutes, 2x/day.

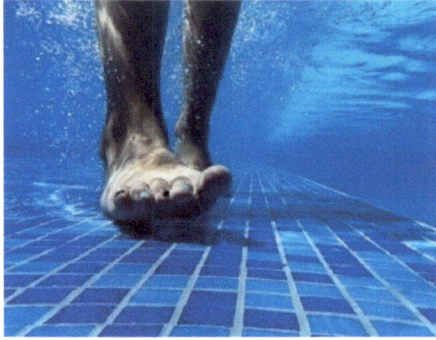

Pool. Walk and perform home exercise in a pool pending your surgical incision is well healed.

5 BALANCE EXERCISES

Exercises to improve **balance**:

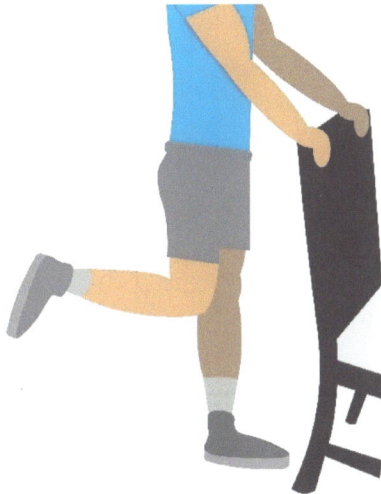

Single Leg Stance. Hold onto stable surface for balance.
Lift one leg from the floor, and balance on the stance leg.
Push down with the big toe of the stance leg and contract
the gluteal and abdominal muscles. Hold 15 seconds.
Perform 3 repetitions, 1x/day.
*Progress from tight grip with hands to light grip to
fingertip touch as able

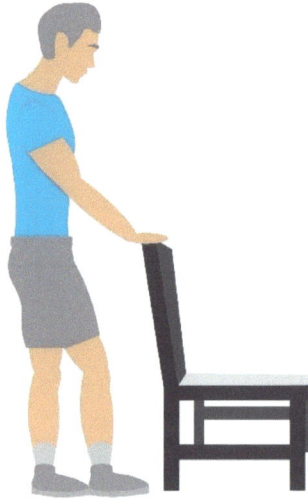

Tandem Stance. Hold onto stable surface for balance as needed. Stand with the toes of one foot touching the heel of the other foot. Push down with the big toes and contract the gluteal and abdominal muscles. Switch foot position, repeat. Hold 15 seconds. Perform 3 repetitions, 1x/day.
*Progress from tight grip with hands to light grip to fingertip touch as able

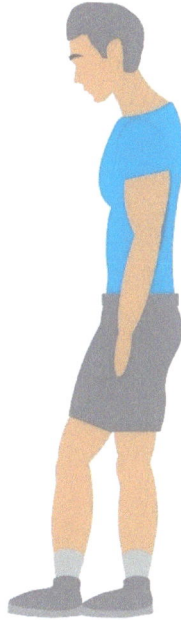

Tandem Walk. Hold on to a stable surface for balance as needed. Walk a straight line of 10 feet with the toes of one foot touching the heel of the other foot. Perform 3 repetitions, 1x/day.

6 GAIT

Normalize gait. Stand up straight, and work toward normalizing gait pattern. Allow the knee to bend during swing phase and work toward improved knee extension during stance phase. Use a step-through pattern versus step-to with walking.

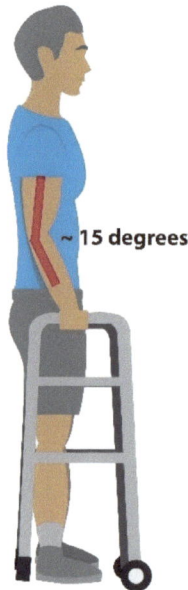

Walker height. Stand up straight with your arms hanging naturally at your sides, the walker handle should be at the level of the crease in your wrist. Your elbow should have ~ 15 degree bend when hand is on handle.

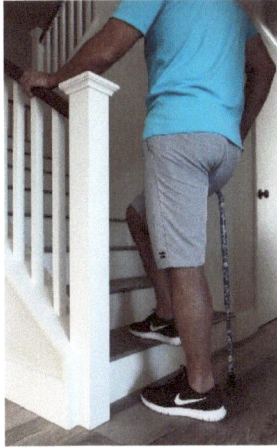

Stairs. Step to pattern on stairs initially with good side leading up, operative side leading down. Progress to reciprocal pattern as pain subsides, and strength improves. Point feet forward, and avoid knock kneed position while ascending and descending stairs.

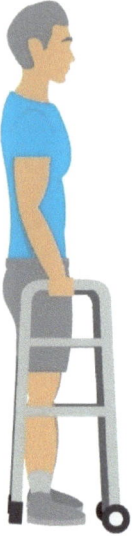

Front Wheel   Four Wheel Walker   Single Point
Walker   Cane

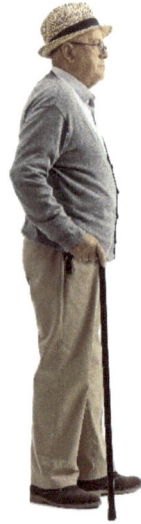

Assistive Device Progression. A walker or front wheel walker is used initially for gait after knee replacement surgery. As leg strength and balance improve, and pain and swelling dissipate, progression to a 4 wheel walker or cane may be appropriate.

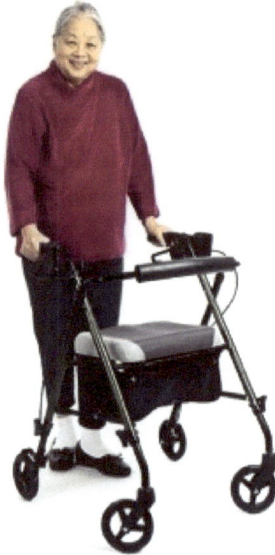

*Use cane in opposite hand of operative leg

7 SWELLING MANAGEMENT

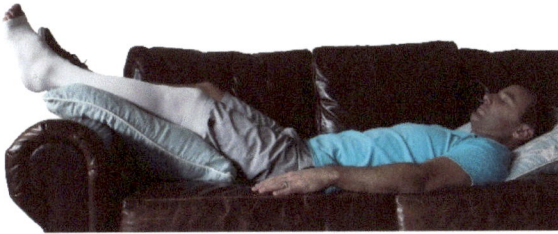

Rest. As you return to your activities of daily living, plan for rest periods throughout the day. While upright, your legs are in a dependent position, and after prolonged upright activity swelling can increase. Rest as needed with the leg elevated to reduce swelling.

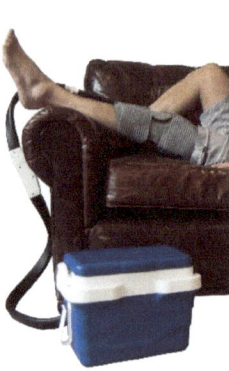 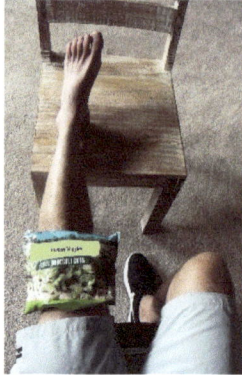 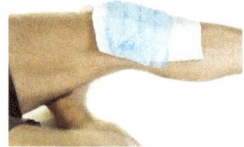

Ice Machine   Frozen Vegetables   Cold Pack

Ice. Cryotherapy, or cold therapy, can be used to reduce pain and swelling after surgery. Ice machines, bags of frozen vegetables, ice bags, or cold packs can be utilized. 20 minute application as needed throughout the day.

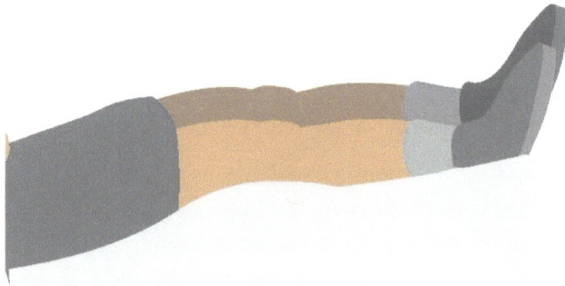

Elevation. Elevation of the swollen limb can reduce swelling. A supine or recumbent position with the leg elevated above your heart is optimal.

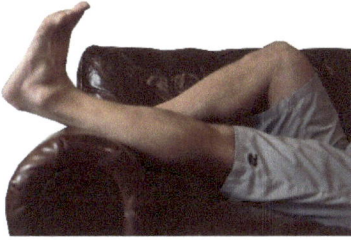

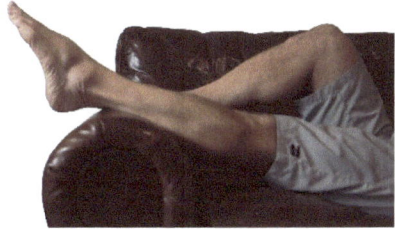

Elevated Ankle Pumps. Elevate the leg above the heart. Pump foot up and down (point and flex). Perform 15 repetitions, 3x/day.

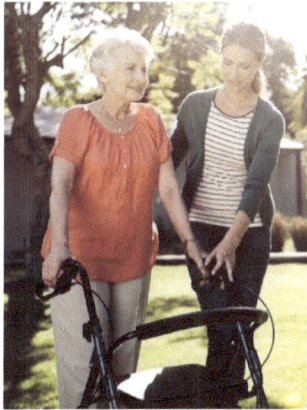

Activity. Activity and exercise require muscle contraction which assists with blood flow return to the heart. Walking and performing home exercises will assist with swelling reduction.

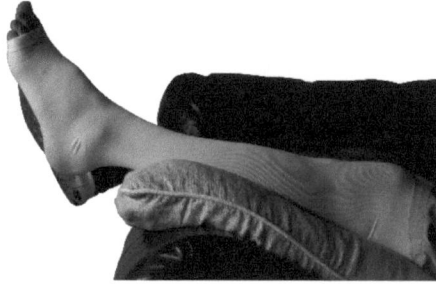

Compression. Graduated compression hose or compression socks can be useful to decrease swelling.

8 PRECAUTIONS

Fall Prevention. Remove throw rugs, extension cords, and any other floor clutter in the home. Ensure railings and grab bars are sturdy prior to use. Use extra caution during mobility if pets or young children are in the vicinity. Ensure your assistive device (walker or cane) is sturdy, and adjusted to the appropriate height. To adjust walker or cane height: Stand up straight with your arms hanging naturally at your sides, the walker or cane handle should be at the level of the crease in your wrist. Your elbow should have ~ 15 degree bend when hand is on handle. Wear non slip footwear.

Infection. Signs and symptoms of infection can include fever, chills, night sweats, wound drainage, fatigue, increased redness, warmth, swelling, or increased pain of the knee or incision area. Report any signs or symptoms of infection to your doctor.

Wound Care. Infection prevention and wound closure are goals for your surgical incision. Ensure the wound stays clean and dry. Comply with follow up appointments after surgery for wound checks and dressing changes. Follow your doctor's protocol for bathing/showering.

Medication. Ensure your doctor has a complete and up to date list of any medication you were taking prior to surgery, including dosage. Follow pre and post operative medication instructions. Monitor and report to your doctor any adverse reaction. When weaning from prescription pain medication, increased use of ice and elevation can be utilized for pain management. Talk to your doctor about over the counter medications as needed.

Deep Vein Thrombosis. A deep vein thrombosis or DVT is a blood clot in a large vein, usually in the legs. Risk of DVT increases with surgery and subsequent prolonged periods of rest or immobility. Other risk factors of DVT can include history of DVT, blood disorders, vascular insufficiency, diabetes, hormone treatment, dehydration, obesity, inflammatory conditions, age, smoking, and cancer treatment. A DVT can present with no signs or symptoms at all, or may present as redness, swelling or pain usually in the calf muscle area. Comply with follow up appointments with your doctor and report any signs or symptoms of DVT.

Pulmonary Embolism. A pulmonary embolism or PE is a blockage in a lung artery. PE can occur if a piece of deep vein thrombosis or DVT has broken off and travelled through the vascular system to lodge in the lungs. Signs and symptoms of a PE are shortness of breath, chest pain, rapid or irregular heart rate, dizziness, excessive sweating, fever, bluish discoloration of lips, mouth, hands or feet, cough, or bloody sputum. PE is a medical emergency. Seek medical attention immediately if signs or symptoms of PE are present.

Range of Motion. Check with your doctor and physical therapist what your expected range of motion goals are. Full knee extension or straight 0 degrees, and flexion or bend of = to or >120 degrees is expected after knee replacement. Avoid sleeping with any pillows under the knee. Perform home exercises 2-3x/day, and comply with swelling management techniques.

9 RETURN TO ACTIVITY

Driving.   Check with your doctor for return to driving readiness. You will need to abstain from pain medication, have sufficient leg strength, and the ability to move your right foot from gas to brake pedal quickly; left foot operating clutch as needed.

Work.   Check with your doctor regarding return to work readiness.   Plan to continue with swelling management techniques.

Walking.   Whether outdoors, or on a treadmill, a post-operative walking program is an ideal exercise to return to. Take seated rest breaks as needed to avoid exhaustion, and continue with swelling management.

Aquatic Exercise.   Once your incision is well-healed, aquatic exercise is an ideal way to improve your endurance and activity tolerance.   Walking and performing exercise in a pool enables you to move your joints in an unweighted environment.

Cycling. Stationary cycling is an ideal way to exercise the lower extremities, and cardiovascular system. If you plan to return to cycling outdoors, check with your doctor. You would need the ability to mount/dismount the bicycle safely, stop and start readily, and have sufficient knee range of motion to pedal a full revolution (a bend of at least 110 degrees).

Golfing. Check with your doctor regarding readiness for return to golf. Work up to full play by putting and chipping, initially. Use a cart and play a short course until ready to return to a full course.

High Impact Activity. Check with your doctor regarding return to high impact activity such as running, tennis, basketball, and aerobics.

10 FAQ

Q: What are knee replacement parts made of?
A: Materials used can include cobalt-chromium, titanium and zirconium alloys, oxinium, tantalum, polyethylene, and polymethyl methacrylate (bonding agent).

Q: Will my knee replacement parts set off the metal detector in airport security?
A: If you have metal in your joint replacement, yes. A TSA notification card can be obtained to hand to security screeners, though you are not exempt from all screening.

Q: How long until I am back on my feet?
A: Pending no complications, expect return to activity by three to six months.

Q: Will I be using a continuous passive motion (CPM) machine after surgery?
A: Your surgeon will determine if you are to use a CPM machine after surgery.

Q: What is a manipulation?
A: A manipulation under anesthesia (MUA) is a technique to mobilize a joint passively when scar tissue has compromised motion.

Q: Will I need a manipulation?
A: The need for manipulation under anesthesia (MUA) after knee replacement surgery is not a desirable outcome. To avoid the need for MUA, comply with post-operative instructions from your doctor and physical therapist to regain range of motion.

Q: Will my legs be the same length after surgery?
A: Your surgeon will select the type and size of prosthesis that is appropriate for you. If limb length discrepancy is a post-surgical problem, notify your surgeon, physical therapist and orthotist.

ABOUT THE AUTHOR

Susan Yovanno is a licensed Doctor of Physical Therapy and board certified Orthopedic Clinical Specialist in California. She treats orthopedic outpatients, and her passion is to educate people to be involved in their own health care and improve their ability to move.